P9-CQX-956

Quick Guide
to HIPAA

for the
Physician's Office

Brenda K. Burton, Director
MEDEXTEND
Fayetteville, GA 30215
http://medextend.com

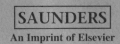

SAUNDERS
An Imprint of Elsevier

SAUNDERS
An Imprint of Elsevier

11830 Westline Industrial Drive
St. Louis, Missouri 63146

QUICK GUIDE TO HIPAA FOR THE PHYSICIAN'S OFFICE   ISBN   0-7216-3935-6
Copyright © 2004, Elsevier. All rights reserved.

Acquisitions Editor: Susan Cole
Project Manager: Peggy Fagen
Designer: Paula Ruckenbrod

Printed in the United States of America

Last digit is the print number: 9 8 7 6 5 4

Health Insurance Portability and Accountability Act (HIPAA)

The U.S. health care system has undergone rapid change with regard to the separate issues of privacy, security, and claims processing over the past decade. Any business that is involved with the health care industry must conform their practices to follow the principles and practices as identified by state and federal agencies. These efforts are generally identified as **compliance.** The professional elements include regulations and recommendations to protect individuals, streamline processes, and increase system-wide stability. A compliance strategy provides a standardized process for handling business functions, leading to consistent and effective management and staff performance. Failure to comply with mandates leads to sanctions and fines from state and federal agencies; failure to follow guidelines potentially results in more fraud and abuse in the claims reimbursement cycle.

The *Health Insurance Portability and Accountability Act* of 1996 (**HIPAA**), Public Law 104-191, will have significant impact on both individuals and health care providers over the next several years. There are two provisions of HIPAA, *Title I: Insurance Reform* and *Title II: Administrative Simplification*. HIPAA projects long-term benefits that include lowered administrative costs, increased accuracy of data, increased patient and customer satisfaction, and reduced revenue cycle time, ultimately improving financial management.

TITLE I: HEALTH INSURANCE REFORM

The primary purpose of HIPAA Title I, *Insurance Reform* is to provide continuous insurance coverage for workers and their insured dependents when they change or lose jobs. This aspect of HIPAA affects individuals as consumers, not particularly as patients. Previously, when an employee left or lost a job and changed insurance coverage, a "preexisting" clause prevented or limited coverage for certain medical conditions. HIPAA now limits the use of preexisting condition exclusions, prohibits discrimination for past or present poor health, and guarantees certain employers and individuals the right to purchase new health insurance coverage after losing a job. Additionally,

This paper is intended to promote awareness. It is not all-encompassing in regard to HIPAA and OIG compliance. It is not intended to replace policy and procedures manuals and similar policy documents.
Definitions from the *Federal Register* are excerpts, used for ease of understanding.

HIPAA allows renewal of health insurance coverage regardless of an individual's health condition that is covered under the particular policy.

TITLE II: ADMINISTRATIVE SIMPLIFICATION

The goals of HIPAA Title II, *Administrative Simplification,* focus on the health care practice setting and are intended to reduce administrative costs and burdens. This is being accomplished by standardizing the exchange of health care data, which will, in itself, increase the use and efficiency of computer-to-computer methods transactions. Additional provisions are meant to ensure the privacy and security of an individual's health data. Standardizing electronic transmissions of administrative and financial information will reduce the number of forms and methods used in the claims processing cycle and reduce the nonproductive effort that goes into processing paper or nonstandard electronic claims.

The two parts of the Administrative Simplification provisions are as follows:

1. Development and implementation of standardized electronic transactions using common sets of descriptors (i.e., Standard Code Sets). These must be used to represent health care concepts and procedures when performing health-related financial and administrative activities electronically (i.e., Standard Transactions).

   • Electronic Health Transaction Standards (specific format information transmitted using Electronic Data Interchange)

   • Standard Code Sets (identify diagnosis, procedures, services, drugs, and supplies)

   • Unique Identifiers for Providers, Employers, Health Plans, and Patients (numeric and alphanumeric strings attached to identify a particular provider, employer, etc.)

Examples of Administrative Information	Examples of Financial Information
Referral Certification and Authorization for Services	Healthcare Claim Submission for Services
Enrollment/Disenrollment of Individual into Health Plan	Process Health Plan Premium Payment
Health Plan Eligibility	Check Status of a Previously Submitted Claim
	Healthcare Payment and Remittance Advice
	Coordination of Benefits

2. Implementation of privacy and security procedures to prevent the misuse of health information by ensuring confidentiality.

   • Privacy and confidentiality

   • Security of health information

Administrative simplification has created uniform sets of standards that protect and place limits on how confidential health information can be used. For years, health care providers have locked medical records in file cabinets and refused to share patient health information. Patients now have specific rights regarding how their health information is used and disclosed because federal and state laws regulate the protection of an individual's privacy. Knowledge and attention to the rights of patients are important to the compliance endeavor in a health care practice. Providers are entrusted with health information and are expected to recognize when certain health information can be used or disclosed. Patients have the legal right to request (1) access and amendments to their health records, (2) an accounting of those who have received their health information, and (3) restrictions on who can access their health records. Understanding the parameters concerning these rights is crucial to complying with HIPAA.

Health care providers and their employer can be held accountable for using or disclosing patient health information inappropriately. HIPAA regulations will be enforced, as clearly stated by the U.S. government. The revolution of HIPAA will take time to understand and implement correctly, but once the standards are in place both within the practice setting and across the sector, greater benefits will be appreciated by the health care provider, staff, and patients.

Compliance Deadlines

Before a rule (or law) becomes final, a preliminary draft is published in the *Federal Register* (FR) as a Notice of Proposed Rule Making (NPRM). As defined by the U.S. Government Printing Office, "The *Federal Register* is the official daily publication for Rules, Proposed Rules, and Notices of Federal agencies and organizations, as well as Executive Orders and other Presidential Documents." After the comment period, the NPRM is usually modified to reflect the consensus of the comments and the best judgment of the staff. Generally, once final rules are published, there is a 2 year plus 60 day period before the rule becomes effective. Upcoming legislation with further mandates from HIPAA will bring more changes. Specific rules and their deadlines at this time are as follows:

- Transactions and Code Set Standards: October 16, 2003

- Medicare Requirement to Submit Electronic Claims: Interim final rule effective October 16, 2003. Final rule estimated to publish September 2006

- Privacy: April 14, 2003

- Standard Unique Employer Identifier: July 30, 2004

- Security Standards: April 21, 2005

- Standard Unique Health Care Provider Identifier: May 23, 2007

- Standard Unique Health Plan Payer Identifier: Proposed rule estimated to publish November 2004

- Standard Unique Individual Identifier: Halted due to privacy concerns

- Standard Claims Attachments: Notice of Proposed Rule Making estimated to publish November 2004

Defining Roles and Relationships: Key Terms

HIPAA legislation required the *U.S. Department of Health and Human Services* (**HHS**) to establish national standards and identifiers for electronic transactions as well as implement privacy and security standards. In regard to HIPAA, **Secretary** refers to the HHS Secretary or any officer or employee of HHS to whom the authority involved has been delegated.

The *Centers for Medicare and Medicaid* (**CMS**) will enforce the insurance portability and transaction and code set requirements of HIPAA. This federal organization was known as the Health Care Financing Administration (HCFA) until June 2001.

The *Office of Civil Rights* (**OCR**) will enforce privacy standards.

A **covered entity** transmits health information in *electronic form* in connection with a *transaction* covered by HIPAA. The covered entity may be (1) a health plan such as Blue Cross/Blue Shield, (2) a health care clearinghouse through which claims are submitted, or (3) a health care provider such as the primary care physician.

A **business associate** is a person who, on behalf of the covered entity, performs or assists in the performance of a function or activity involving the use or disclosure of individually identifiable health information, including claims processing or administration, data analysis, processing or administration, utilization review, quality assurance, billing, benefit management, practice management, and repricing. For example, if a provider practice contracts with an outside billing company to manage its claims and accounts receivable, the billing company would be a business associate of the provider (the covered entity).

Electronic media refer to the mode of electronic transmission, including the following:

- Internet (wide open)

- Extranet or private network using Internet technology to link business parties

- Leased phone or dial-up phone lines, including fax modems (speaking over phone not considered an electronic transmission)

- Transmissions that are physically moved from one location to another using magnetic tape, disk, or compact disk media

A **health care provider** is a provider of medical or health services and any other person or organization who furnishes, bills, or is paid for health care in the normal course of business.

Privacy and security officers oversee the HIPAA-related functions. These individuals may or may not be employees of a particular health care practice. A *privacy officer* or *privacy official* (**PO**) is designated to help the provider remain in compliance by setting policies and procedures in place, training and managing the staff regarding HIPAA and patient rights, and generally functioning as the contact person for questions and complaints. A *security officer* protects the computer and networking systems within the practice and implements protocols such as password assignment, back up procedures, firewalls, virus protection, and contingency planning for emergencies.

A **transaction** refers to the transmission of information between two parties to carry out financial or administrative activities related to health care. These information transmissions include the following:

1. Health care claims or equivalent encounter information

2. Health care payment and remittance advice

3. Coordination of benefits

4. Health care claim status

5. Enrollment and disenrollment in a health plan

6. Eligibility for a health plan

7. Health plan premium payments

8. Referral certification and authorization

9. First report of injury

10. Health claim attachments

11. Other transactions that the Secretary may prescribe by regulation

TPO refers to *treatment, payment,* and *health care operations.*

Application to practice setting. The previous "roles" create relationships that guide the health care provider and the practice. A *health care provider* can include a nurse practitioner, social worker, chiropractor, radiologist, or dentist; HIPAA does not affect only medical physicians. The health care provider is designated as a HIPAA-mandated Covered Entity under certain conditions. It is important to remember that health care providers who transmit any health information in electronic form in connection with a HIPAA transaction are covered entities. Electronic form or media can include floppy disk, compact disk (CD), or file transfer protocol (FTP) over the Internet. Voice-over-modem faxes, meaning a phone line, are not considered electronic media, although a fax from a computer (e.g., WinFax program) is considered an electronic medium.

HIPAA requires the designation of a PO to develop and implement the organization's policies and procedures. The PO for an organization may hold another position within the practice or may not be an employee of the practice at all. Often, the PO is a contracted professional and available to the practice through established means of contact.

HIPAA FOCUS

Simply put, if a health care provider either transmits directly or utilizes a "business associate" (e.g., billing company or clearinghouse) to transmit information electronically for any of the transactions listed, the health care provider is a "covered entity" and must comply with HIPAA.

The business associate often is considered an extension of the provider practice. If an office function is outsourced with use or disclosure of individually identifiable health information, the organization that is acting on behalf of the health care provider is considered a business associate. For example, if the office's medical transcription is performed by an outside service, the transcription service is a Business Associate of the Covered Entity (the health care provider/practice).

HIPAA privacy regulations as a federal mandate will apply unless the state laws are contrary or more stringent with regard to privacy. **State preemption,** a complex technical issue not within the scope of the health care provider's role, refers to instances when state law takes precedence over federal law. The PO will determine when the need for preemption arises.

Privacy Rule: Confidentiality and Protected Health Information

> What I may see or hear in the course of the treatment or even outside of the treatment in regard to the life of men, which on no account one must spread abroad, I will keep to myself holding such things shameful to be spoken about.
>
> *Hippocrates, 400 BC*

The Hippocratic Oath, federal and state regulations, professional standards, and ethics all address patient privacy. Because current technology allows easy access to health care information, HIPAA imposes new requirements for health care providers. Since computers have become indispensable for the health care office, confidential health data have been sent across networks, e-mailed over the Internet, and even exposed by hackers, with few safeguards taken to protect data and prevent information from being intercepted or lost. With the implementation of standardizing electronic transactions of health care information, the use of technologies will pose new risks for privacy and security. These concerns were addressed under HIPAA, and regulations now closely govern how the industry handles its electronic activities.

Privacy is the condition of being secluded from the presence or view of others. **Confidentiality** is using discretion in keeping secret information. Integrity plays an important part in the health care setting. Staff members of a health care organization need a good understanding of HIPAA's basic requirements and must be committed to protecting the privacy and rights of the practice's patients.

Disclosure means the release, transfer, provision of access to, or divulging in any other manner of information outside the entity holding the information. An example of a "disclosure" would be if you give information to the hospital's outpatient surgery center about a patient you are scheduling for a procedure.

Individually identifiable health information (**IIHI**) is any part of an individual's health information, including demographic information (e.g., address, date of birth) collected from the individual that is created or received by a covered entity. This information relates to the individual's past, present, or future physical or mental health or condition; the provision of health care to the individual; or the past, present, or future payment for the provision of health care. IIHI data identify the individual or establish a reasonable basis to believe the information can be used to identify the individual. For example, if you as health care provider are talking to an insurance representative, you will likely give information such as the patient's date of birth and last name. These pieces of information would make it reasonably easy to identify the patient. If you are talking to a pharmaceutical representative about a drug assistance program that covers a new pill for heartburn, and you only say that your practice has a patient living in your town who is indigent and has stomach problems, you are not divulging information that would identify the patient.

Protected health information (**PHI**) refers to IIHI that is transmitted by electronic media, maintained in electronic form, or transmitted or maintained in any other form or medium. PHI does not include IHII in education records covered by the Family Educational Right and Privacy Act.

Traditionally, there has been focus on protecting paper medical records and documentation that held patient's health information, such as laboratory results and radiology reports. HIPAA Privacy Regulation expands these protections to apply to PHI. The individual's health information is protected regardless of the type of medium in which it is maintained. This includes paper, the health care provider's computerized practice management and billing system, spoken words, and x-ray films.

Use means the sharing, employment, application, utilization, examination, or analysis of IHII within an organization that holds such information. When a patient's billing record is accessed to review the claim submission history, the individual's health information is in "use."

HIPAA imposes requirements to protect not only disclosure of PHI outside of the organization but also for internal uses of health information. PHI may not be used or disclosed without permission of the patient or someone authorized to act on behalf of the patient, unless the use or disclosure is specifically required or permitted by the regulation (e.g., TPO). The two types of disclosure required by HIPAA Privacy Rule are to the individual who is the subject of the PHI and to the Secretary or DHHS to investigate compliance with the rule.

Privacy Rule: Patient Rights under HIPAA

Patients are granted the following federal rights that allow them to be informed about PHI and to control how their PHI is used and disclosed:

1. Right to Notice of Privacy Practices

2. Right to request restrictions on certain uses and disclosures of PHI

3. Right to request confidential communications

4. Right to access (inspect and obtain a copy of) PHI

5. Right to request an amendment of PHI

6. Right to receive an accounting of disclosures of PHI

Right to Notice of Privacy Practices. Under HIPAA, patients are entitled to receive the written Notice of Privacy Practices (NPP) of their provider at the first appointment. The NPP outlines the individual's rights and covered entity's legal duties in regard to PHI. The NPP must be provided and written in "plain language" and the staff must make a reasonable "best effort" to obtain a signature from the patient acknowledging receipt. This can be recorded simply as signing a label on the inside cover of the chart. The front desk reception area is an ideal location for distribution of the NPP to the patient with the registration sheet and other required forms. If the patient cannot or will not sign, a staff member can sign and date the receipt for them. An NPP will be tailored to each organization and must explain the following:

- How PHI may be used and disclosed by the organization
- Health provider duties to protect PHI
- Patient rights regarding PHI
- How complaints may be filed with the office and HHS if the patient believes his or her privacy rights have been violated
- Who to contact for further information (usually the PO)
- Effective date of the NPP

As a health care provider, you may have already seen these notices posted at your pharmacy or had to sign an acknowledgment that you read a copy of the NPP at your personal physician's office. Your patients must have ready access to your organization's NPP. This Notice must be posted prominently in the office (e.g., on the wall by the reception desk) and must be available in paper form for patients who request it. If your office has a website, the Notice must be posted prominently there as well. HIPAA states that covered entities may not require individuals to waive their rights "as a condition of the provision of treatment or payment."

Right to request restrictions on certain uses and disclosures of PHI. Patients do have the right to ask for restrictions on how your office uses and discloses PHI for TPO. Patients may have items in their previous medical history that are not applicable to the current disclosure and may even cause the patient embarrassment; patients may request that this PHI not be disclosed (e.g., a patient had a successfully treated STD many years before and requests that, whenever possible, this material not be disclosed). The covered entity is not required to agree to these requests but must have a process to review the requests, accept and review any appeal, and give a sound reason for not agreeing to the request. If agreed upon, however, the restrictions must be documented and followed. Such restrictions may be tracked by flagging the patient's medical chart that a restriction applies or by using a pop-up note in the practice management software. There must be an implemented procedure in place to check for any restrictions before PHI is disclosed.

A practice may disclose confidential information in certain situations *without* a written authorization from the patient (e.g., reporting communicable diseases, reporting about victims of abuse, and for law enforcement purposes). You can ask your PO or refer to the *Policy and Procedure Manual* for clarification when disclosures are permissible.

In addition, unless a patient has requested that such disclosures *not* occur and the provider has agreed, health information may be disclosed to a family member, relative, close friend, or any other person identified by the patient.

HIPAA FOCUS

In regard to the *patient's right to request restrictions on certain uses and disclosures of PHI,* you will find key terms addressed in the NPP that apply to this right.

- **Minimum Necessary.** Privacy regulations require that use or disclosure of only the minimum amount of information necessary to fulfill the intended purpose be permitted. There are some exceptions to this rule. You do not need to limit PHI for disclosures in regard to health care providers for treatment, the patient, HHS for investigations of compliance with HIPAA, or as required by law.

  Minimum necessary determinations for *uses of PHI* must be determined within each organization, and reasonable efforts must be made to limit access to only the minimum amount of information needed by identified staff members. In smaller offices, employees may have multiple job functions. If a medical assistant helps with the patient exam, documents vital signs, and then collects the patient's co-pay at the reception area, the assistant will likely access clinical and billing records. Simple procedure and policy (P&P) about appropriate access to PHI may be sufficient to satisfy the Minimum Necessary requirement. Larger organizations may have specific restrictions on who should have access to different types of PHI, because staff members tend to have a more targeted job role. Remain knowledgeable about your office's policy regarding Minimum Necessary. If you are strictly scheduling appointments, you may not need access to the clinical record. An x-ray technician will likely not need to access the patient billing records.

Minimum Necessary Determinations for *disclosures of PHI* are distinguished by two categories within the Privacy Rule:

  1. For disclosures made on a routine and recurring basis, you may implement policies and procedures, or standard protocols, for what will be disclosed. These disclosures would be common in your practice. Examples may include disclosures for workers' compensation claims or school physical forms.
  2. For other disclosures that would be considered non-routine, criteria should be established for determining the Minimum Necessary amount of PHI and to review each request for disclosure on an individual basis. There will be a staff member (e.g., PO, Medical Records Supervisor) likely assigned to determine this situation when need arises.

As a general rule, remember that you must limit your requests to access PHI to the Minimum Necessary to accomplish the task for which you will need the information.

- **De-identification of Confidential Information.** Other requirements relating to uses and disclosures of PHI include health information that does not identify an individual or leaves no reasonable basis to believe that the information can be used to identify an individual. This "de-identified" information is no longer individually identifiable health information (IIHI). Most providers will never have the need to de-identify patient information, and the requirements for de-identifying PHI are lengthy. The regulations give specific directions on how to ensure all pieces of necessary information are removed to fit the definition. De-identified information is not subject to the privacy regulations because it does not specifically identify an individual.

Continued

- **Marketing** refers to communicating about a product or service where the goal is to encourage patients to purchase or use the product or service. For instance, a dermatologist may advertise for a discount on facial cream when you schedule a dermabrasion treatment. You will likely not be involved in marketing, but keep in mind the general rule that PHI (including names and addresses) cannot be used for marketing purposes without specific authorization of the patient. Sending appointment reminders and general news updates about your organization and the services you provide would not be considered marketing and would not require patient authorization.
- **Fundraising.** Again, you will likely not be involved in fundraising activities, but HIPAA allows demographic information and dates of care to be used for fundraising purposes without patient authorization. The disclosure of any additional information requires patient authorization. Your organization's NPP will state that patients may receive fundraising materials and are given the opportunity to opt out of receiving future solicitations.

Right to request confidential communications. A patient can request to receive confidential communications by alternative means or at an alternative location. For example, a patient may ask that the health care provider call the patient at work rather than at the residence or patients may request that their test results be sent to them in writing rather than by phone. It is the patient's right to request such alternative methods of communication, and the health care office must accommodate *reasonable* requests. This can become a serious issue, especially in cases of domestic violence when the individual is at risk for physical harm within the home environment. The patient does not need to explain the reason for the request. The health care office must have a process in place both to evaluate requests and appeals and to respond to the patient.

Patients may be required by the office to make their request in writing. Documenting such requests in writing with the patient's signature is an effective way to protect the practice's compliance endeavors. The office may even condition the agreement by arranging for payment of any additional costs from the patient that the request has created. For example, the patient asks that all correspondence be sent by registered mail; this request may be able to be honored without significant additional staff time but the patient should expect to incur the actual additional mailing costs.

Right to access PHI (inspect and obtain a copy). A patient has the right to access, inspect, and obtain a copy of his or her confidential health information. Privacy regulations allow the provider to require the patient make the request for access in writing. Generally, a request must be acted on within 30 days. A reasonable, cost-based fee for copies of PHI may only include the costs for the following:

- Supplies and labor for copying
- Postage when mailed

- Preparing a summary of the PHI if the patient has agreed to this instead of complete access

This "fee" for copying varies widely by state and each provider should be aware of the state allowances and conform their fee to that which gives most relief to the patient. The HIPAA-determined fee applies <u>only</u> to fees for copies to patients and not copies for other required or allowed disclosures, e.g. subpoenas. The fee structures for other disclosures are often set by state law. If you are a staff member involved in applying fees for copying, you should seek guidance from your Privacy Officer.

Under HIPAA Privacy Regulation, patients do not have the right to access the following:

- Psychotherapy notes

- Information compiled in reasonable anticipation of, or for use in, legal proceedings

- Information exempted from disclosure under the Clinical Laboratory Improvements Amendment (CLIA)

The office may deny patient access for the above reasons without giving the patient the right to review the denial. Also, if the PHI was obtained from an individual other than a health care provider under a promise of confidentiality, access may be denied if such access would likely reveal the identity of the source. Other circumstances in which an individual may be denied access will be detailed in the practice's policy manual.

If the health care provider has determined that the patient would be endangered (or cause danger to another person) from accessing the confidential health information, access may be denied. In this case the patient has the right to have the denial reviewed by another licensed professional who did not participate in the initial denial decision.

HIPAA specifically excludes from Psychotherapy Notes information about medication management, start and stop times of sessions, frequency and type of treatment provided, results of testing, and summaries of diagnosis, treatment plan, symptoms, prognosis, and progress to date. These are, however, PHI. Psychotherapy notes are not stored in the general client record, nor are Personal Notes.

HIPAA affords psychotherapy notes more protection—most notably from third-party payers—than they'd been given in the past. Under HIPAA, disclosure of psychotherapy notes requires more than just generalized consent; it requires patient authorization—or specific permission—to release this sensitive information (e.g. to a third party).

Though the privacy rule does afford patients the right to access and inspect their health records, psychotherapy notes are treated differently: Patients do *not* have the right to obtain a copy of these under HIPAA. Under the new law, psychologists can decide whether to release their psychotherapy notes to patients, unless patients would have access to their psychotherapy notes under state law. If a psychologist denies a patient access to these notes, the denial isn't subject to a review process, as it is with other records.

There is a catch in the psychotherapy notes provision. HIPAA's definition of psychotherapy notes explicitly states that these notes are kept separate from the rest of an individual's record. So, if a psychologist keeps this type of information in a patient's general chart, or if it's not distinguishable as separate from the rest of the record, access to the information doesn't require specific patient authorization.

State law must be considered since, in all cases where state law is more strict or gives the patient more access to information, state law takes precedence.

Right to request amendment of PHI. Patients have the right to request that their PHI be amended. As with the other requests, the provider may require the request be in writing. The provider must have a process to accept and review both the request and any appeal in a timely fashion. The health care provider may deny this request in the following circumstances:

- The provider who is being requested to change the PHI is not the creator of the information (e.g., office has records sent by referring physician).

- The PHI is believed to be accurate and complete as it stands in the provider's records.

- The information is not required to be accessible to the patient (see Right to access PHI).

Generally, the office must respond to a patient's request for amendment within 60 days. If a request is denied, the patient must be informed in writing of the reason for the denial. The patient must also be given the opportunity to file a statement of disagreement. These rules are complex in regard to steps of appeal, rebuttal, and documentation that must be provided if a request for amendment is denied. The PO will instruct providers on additional responsibilities if they are directly involved in this process.

Right to receive an accounting of disclosures of PHI. Providers should maintain a log of disclosures of PHI, either paper or within the organization's computer system of all disclosures other than those made for TPO, facility directories, and some national security and law enforcement agencies. The process for providing an accounting should be outlined in the practice's policy manual. Patients may request an accounting (or tracking) of disclosures of their confidential information and are granted the right to receive

HIPAA FOCUS

HIPAA regulations recognize that certain kinds of mental health information need to be protected more than other types of information. Under HIPAA, psychotherapy notes are defined as "notes recorded in any medium by a mental health professional documenting or analyzing the contents of conversation during a private counseling session." These notes, which capture the psychologist's impressions about the patient and can contain information that is inappropriate for a medical record, are similar to what psychologists have historically referred to as "process notes."

this accounting once a year without charge. Additional accountings may be assessed a cost-based fee.

These accountings are only required to start on April 14, 2003, when privacy regulations became enforceable. Items to be documented must include the following:

- Date of disclosure

- Name of the entity or person who received the PHI, including their address if known

- Brief description of the PHI disclosed

- Brief statement of the purpose of the disclosure

The patient is entitled to one accounting per year free of charge. Additional accountings may be assessed a cost-based fee.

HIPAA FOCUS

In summary, patients have the right to:
- Be informed of the organization's privacy practices by receiving a Notice of Privacy Practices (NPP).
- Have their information kept confidential and secure.
- Obtain a copy of their health record.
- Request to have their health records amended.
- Request special considerations in communication.
- Restrict unauthorized access to their confidential health information.

HIPAA FOCUS

Health care providers and staff will likely not be reading the *Federal Register* and thus will want to familiarize themselves with the general forms used in their practice setting. They should be aware of the following:
- **Written acknowledgement.** After providing the patient with the NPP, a "good faith" effort must be made to obtain written acknowledgment of the patient receiving the document. If the patient refuses to sign or is unable to sign, this must be documented in the patient record.
- **Authorization forms.** Use and disclosure of PHI is permissible for TPO because the NPP describes how PHI is used for these purposes. The health care provider is required to obtain signed authorization to use or disclose health information for situations beyond the TPO. This is a protection for the practice. Providers must learn about the particular "authorization" forms used in their office. Psychotherapy notes are handled separately under HIPAA. Such notes have additional protection, specifically, that an authorization for any use of disclosure of psychotherapy notes must be obtained.

Your organization will be expected to handle requests made by patients to exercise their rights. You must know your office's process for dealing with each specific request. With your understanding of HIPAA and your organization's policy manual, you will be guided in procedures specific to your health care practice.

The patients cannot keep their confidential health information from being used for treatment, payment or healthcare operations (TPO) nor may they force amendments to their health record. As you become more acclimated to your organization's policies and procedures regarding the handling of PHI, you will be better able to recognize how your position is an important part in HIPAA compliance.

Organization and Staff Responsibilities in Protecting Patient Rights

The covered entity must implement written *policies and procedures* (**P&P**) that comply with HIPAA standards. P&P are tailored guidelines established to accommodate each health care practice and designed to address PHI. HIPAA requires each practice to implement P&P that comply with privacy and security rules. The office should have a *Policy and Procedure Manual* to train providers and to serve as a resource for situations that need clarification. Revisions in P&P must be made as necessary and appropriate to comply with laws as they change. Documentation must be maintained in written or electronic form and retained for 6 years of its creation or when it was last in effect, whichever is later.

Verification of identity and authority. Prior to any disclosure, you must verify the identity of persons requesting PHI if they are unknown to you. You may request identifying information such as date of birth, social security number, or even a code word stored in your practice management system that is unique to each patient. Public officials may show you badges, credentials, official letterheads, and other legal documents of authority for identification purposes. Additionally, you must verify that the requestor has the right and the need to have the PHI.

Exercising professional judgment will fulfill your verification requirements for most disclosures because you are acting on "good faith" in believing the identity of the individual requesting PHI. It is good practice, when making any disclosure to note, to note the "authority" of the person receiving the PHI and how this was determined. This evidence of due diligence on your part would enforce a needed structure on your staff and dampen any complaints that might arise.

Validating patient permission. Before making any uses or disclosures of confidential health information other than for the purposes of TPO, your office must have appropriate patient permission. Always check for conflicts between various permissions your office may have on file for a given patient. This information should be maintained either in your practice management system or in the medical chart, where it can be easily identified and retrieved.

For example, if a covered entity has agreed to a patient's request to limit how much of the PHI is sent to a consulting physician for treatment, but then received the patient's authorization to disclose the entire medical record to that physician, this would be a conflict. In general, the more restrictive permission would be the deciding factor. Privacy regulations allow resolving conflicting permissions by either obtaining new permission from the patient or by communicating orally or in writing with the patient to determine the patient's preference. Be sure to document any form of communication in writing.

Training. Under HIPAA regulations, a covered entity must train all members of its workforce. This training must include the practice's policies and procedures with respect to PHI as "necessary and appropriate for the members of the workforce to carry out their function within the covered entity." This training will address how your role relates to PHI in your office, and you will be instructed on how to handle confidential information. The PO for your health care practice will likely be the instructor for this type of training. HIPAA training focuses on how to handle confidential information securely in the office, as discussed later.

Safeguards: Ensuring that confidential information is secure. Every covered entity must have appropriate safeguards to ensure the protection of an individual's confidential health information. Such safeguards include administrative, technical, and physical measures that will "reasonably safeguard" PHI from any use or disclosure that violates HIPAA, whether intentional or unintentional.

Example Administrative Safeguard	Example Technical Safeguard	Example Physical Safeguard
Verifying the identity of an individual picking up health records	User name/password required to access patient records from computer	Locked, fireproof filing cabinets for storing paper records

Complaints to Healthcare Practice and Workforce Sanctions. Individuals, both patients and staff, must be provided with a process to make a complaint concerning the P&P of the covered entity. If a violation involves the misuse of PHI, this incident should be reported to the practice's PO. Should there be further cause, the OCR may also be contacted.

Workforce members are subject to appropriate sanctions for failure to comply with the P&P regarding PHI set forth in the office. Types of sanctions applied will vary depending on factors involved with the violation. Sanctions can range from a warning to suspension to termination. This information should be covered in the P&P manual. Written documentation of complaints and sanctions must be prepared with any disposition.

Mitigation. Mitigation means to "alleviate the severity" or "make mild." In reference to HIPAA, the covered entity has an affirmative duty to take reasonable steps in response to breaches. If a breach is discovered, the health care provider is required to mitigate, to the extent possible, any harmful effects of the breach. For example, if you learn you have erroneously sent medical records by fax to an incorrect party, steps should be taken to have the recipient destroy the PHI. Mitigation procedures also include activities of the practice's business associates. Being proactive and responsible by mitigating will reduce the potential for a more disastrous outcome from the breach or violation.

Refraining from intimidating or retaliatory acts. HIPAA privacy regulations prohibit a covered entity from intimidating, threatening, coercing, discriminating against, or otherwise taking retaliatory action against:

- Individuals for exercising HIPAA privacy rights

- Individuals for filing a complaint with HHS or testifying, assisting, or participating in an investigation about the covered entity's privacy practices or reasonably opposing any practice prohibited by the regulation

Transaction and Code Set Regulations: Streamlining Electronic Data Interchange

HIPAA *Transaction and Code Set* (**TCS**) regulation was developed to introduce efficiencies into the health care system. The objectives are to achieve a higher quality of care and to reduce administrative costs by streamlining the processing of routine administrative and financial transactions. HHS has estimated that by implementing TCS, almost $30 billion over 10 years would be saved.

Technology and the use of *Electronic Data Interchange* (**EDI**) has made the processing of transactions more efficient and reduced administrative overhead costs in other industries. EDI is the exchange of data in a standardized format through computer systems. Standardizing transactions and codes sets is required to use EDI effectively, with the implementation of standard formats, procedures, and data content.

TCS regulation requires the implementation of specific standards for transactions and code sets by October 16, 2003. The intent of TCS requirements is to achieve a single standard. As an example in the pre-HIPAA environment, when submitting claims for payment, health care providers have been doing business with insurance payers who require the use of their own version of local code sets (e.g., state Medicaid programs) or identifiers and paper forms. More than 400 versions of a *National Standard Format* (**NSF**) exist to submit a claim for payment. HIPAA will streamline the standards and enable greater administrative efficiencies throughout the health care system. Health care provider offices will benefit from less paperwork, and standardizing data will result in more accurate information and a more efficient organization.

HIPAA standardization actions are similar to using a bank's automatic teller machine (ATM) or the grocery store's self-checkout. A magnetic strip on a bankcard or the bar code on a grocery item can be swiped across a reading mechanism, allowing customers to process a transaction more quickly than with traditional methods. As these methods are adapted, there are benefits to both the end user and the business providing the technology (Table 1).

A provider *is considered a covered entity* under HIPAA in the following circumstances:

- If the provider submits electronic transactions to any payer.

- If the provider submits paper claims to Medicare and has 10 or more employees, the provider is required to convert to electronic transactions (no later than October 16, 2003), and therefore HIPAA compliance is required.

Table 1	*Recognized Benefits of TCS and EDI*
BENEFIT	**RESULT**
More reliable and timely processing of claim data	Fast eligibility evaluation; reduced accounts receivable cycle; industry averages for claim turnarounds are 9-15 days for electronic vs. 30-45 days for paper claims.
Quicker reimbursement from payer	Improves cash flow for the health care organization.
Improved accuracy of data	Decreases processing time, increases data quality, and leads to better reporting.
Easier and more efficient access to information	Improves patient support.
Better tracking of transactions	Facilitates tracking of transactions (i.e., when sent and received), allowing for monitoring (e.g., prompt payments).
Reduction of data entry/manual labor	Electronic transactions facilitate automated processes (e.g., auto payment posting).
Reduction in office expenses	Reduces office supplies, postage, and telephone charges.

Data from HIPAA docs Corporation.

According to CMS, "After October 16, 2003, Electronic Claims will not be processed if they are in a format other than in the HIPAA format. Providers who are not small providers (institutional organizations with fewer than 25 full-time employees or physicians with fewer than 10 full-time employees) must send all claims electronically in the HIPAA format."

A provider *is not considered a covered entity* under HIPAA in the following circumstances:

- If the provider has less than 10 employees and submits claims only on paper to Medicare (not electronic). The provider may continue to submit on paper and therefore is not required to comply with any part of HIPAA (i.e., not required to submit electronically).

- If the provider only submits paper claims until and after April 14, 2003 and does not send claims to Medicare, the provider is not required to comply with sending electronic claims.

Transaction and code set standards. TCS standards by the American National Standards Institute (ANSI) have been adopted for medical transactions. HIPAA transactions are the electronic files in which medical data are compiled to produce a given format. This is *electronic* and not a paper form. The provider cannot print out an "HIPAA claim form" to submit for reimbursement.

In general, *code sets* are the allowable set of codes that anyone could use to enter into a specific space on a form. All health care organizations using electronic transactions will have to use and accept (either directly or through a clearinghouse) the code set systems required under HIPAA that document

specific health care data elements, including medical diagnoses and procedures, drugs, physician services, and medical suppliers. These codes have
already been in common use (required in Medicare and Medicaid claims),
which should help ease the transition to the new transaction requirements.
What has been a standard in the health care industry and recognized by most
payers now is simply *mandated* under HIPAA.

HIPAA standard codes are used in conjunction with the standard electronic
transactions. The health care industry will recognize a standard that will eliminate ambiguity when processing transactions. In turn, this will ultimately
improve the quality of data and result in improved decision making and
reporting in administrative and clinical processes.

Table 2 *HIPAA Medial Code Sets and Elements*

STANDARD CODE SETS	MEDICAL DATA ELEMENTS
International Classification of Diseases, ninth edition, Clinical Modification (ICD-9-CM), Vols 1 and 2 ICD-9-CM replaces DSM-IV.	Diseases Injuries Impairments Other health-related problems and their manifestations Causes of injury, disease, impairment, or other health-related problems
ICD-9-CM, Vol 3	Procedures or other actions taken for diseases, injuries, and impairments on hospital inpatients reported by hospitals, including prevention, diagnosis, treatment, and management
Current Procedural Terminology, fourth edition (CPT-4)	Physician services Physician and occupational therapy services Radiologic procedures Clinical laboratory tests Other medical diagnostic procedures Hearing and vision services Transportation services (e.g., helicopter, ambulance) Other services
Code on Dental Procedures and Nomenclature (CDT)	Dental services
National Drug Codes (NDC) for Retail Pharmacy transactions	Pharmaceuticals Biologics
International Classification of Diseases, tenth edition, Clinical Modification (ICD-10-CM) (diagnosis) ICD-10-PCS (to replace ICD-9-CM, Vol 3 procedural coding system)	Expected to replace ICD-9-CM, but no date has been set.

DSM-IV, *Diagnostic and Statistical Manual of Mental Disorders,* fourth edition.

Medical codes sets are data elements used uniformly to document why patients are seen (diagnosis, ICD-9-CM) and what is done to them during their encounter (procedure, CPT-4 and HCPCS). Each covered entity organization is responsible for implementing the updated codes in a timely manner, using the new HIPAA-mandated TCS codes and deleting old or obsolete ones (Table 2).

HIPAA also provides standards for the complete cycle of administrative transactions and electronic standard formats (Table 3).

Table 3	*HIPAA Transaction Functions and Formats*
STANDARD TRANSACTION FUNCTION	**INDUSTRY FORMAT NAME**
Eligibility Verification/ Response	ASC X12N 270/271 Version 4010
Referral Certification and Authorization	ASC X12N 278 Version 4010
Claims or Equivalent Encounters and Coordination of Benefits	ASC X12N 837 Version 4010. You will become very familiar with this format. The 837P (Professional) will take over the paper CMS-1500 form and the electronic National Standard Format (NSF). The 837I (Institutional) will replace the paper UB-92. 837D (Dental) will be used for dentistry. The encounter for Retail Drug NCPCP v. 32.
Functional Acknowledgment	ASC X12N 997 Version 4010
Health Claim Status Inquiry/Response	ASC X12N 276/277 Version 4010
First Report of Injury (pending)	ASC X12N 148
Payment and Remittance Advice	ASC X12N 835
Health Claims Attachment (pending)	ASC X12 275 & HL7 TBD (No more copying paper attachments and stapling to a CMS-1500)

HIPAA FOCUS

When a patient comes into your office and is treated, his or her confidential health information is collected and put into the computerized practice management system. The services rendered are assigned a standard code from the HIPAA-required *code sets* (e.g., CPT), and the diagnosis is selected from another code set (e.g., ICD-9-CM); much the same as before HIPAA.

When claims are generated for electronic submission, all data collected are compiled and constructed into a HIPAA *standard transaction*. This EDI is recognized across the health care sector in computer systems maintained by providers, the clearinghouses, and insurance payers. The harmony among the covered entities results in a more efficient claim life cycle.

"Out with the old, in with the 837": understanding data requirements.
The health care provider practice and staff will learn about the 837. The role
of the billing specialist in the health care organization will likely not change
drastically because the HIPAA-enabled practice management software system
will produce the required HIPAA standard electronic formats. Additionally,
the continued use of clearinghouses will eliminate much of the confusion for
the organization. However, if you are directly involved in the claims processing procedures, you will need to know the most important items to look for
in regard to HIPAA requirements and situational data and successfully
construct a compliant and payable insurance claim. You will be trained on the
practice management software system on where to put additionally captured
data that have not been collected on the CMS-1500 form or electronic NSF.

In addition to the major code sets (ICD-9 and CPT/HCPCS), several *supporting code sets* encompass both medical and nonmedical data (Table 4). When
constructing a claim, the **supporting code sets are made up of
"Required" and "Situational" data elements, similar to those on
the CMS-1500 paper form.** These supporting code sets are embedded in
the data elements identified by the HIPAA standard electronic formats. You
will not need to know all these specific codes, but it will be helpful to know
they do exist, especially if you are active in the claims-processing procedures.
When reviewing reports from the clearinghouse or the insurance payer, you
may have to correct claims that were rejected for not having correct data
elements.

Required refers to data elements that must used to be in compliance with a
HIPAA standard transaction. Conversely, *situational* means that the item
depends on the data content or context. For example, a baby's birth weight is
obviously "situational" when submitting a claim for the delivery of the
infant. Another situational data element would be the last menstrual period
(LMP) when a female is pregnant. Determining the required and situational
data elements not currently collected for the CMS-1500 claim or NSF electronic format can be quite complex; you will learn this process when you are
in the office performing claims-processing duties. In addition to other data
elements required under HIPAA TCS, examples include the following:

- *Taxonomy codes.* Provider specialty codes assigned to each health care
  provider. Common taxonomy codes include "general practice
  203BG0000Y," "family practice 203BF10100Y," and "nurse practitioner
  363L00000N."

- *Patient account number.* To be assigned to every claim.

- *Relationship to patient.* Expanded to 25 different relationships, including
  indicators such as "grandson," "adopted child," "mother," and "life partner."

- *Facility code value.* Facility-related element that identifies the place of
  service, with at least 29 to choose from, including "office," "ambulance
  air or water," and "end-stage renal disease treatment facility."

- *Patient signature source code.* Indicates how the patient or subscriber signatures were obtained for authorization and how signatures are retained

by the provider. Codes include letters such as **B** for "signed signature authorization form or forms for both HCFA-15—claim form block 12 and block 13 are on file" and **P** for "signature generated by provider because the patient was not physically present for services."

Grouping of information for 837P. Because the 837P is an electronic format and not a paper form, data collected to construct and submit a claim are grouped by levels. Again, it is important for claims-processing staff to know the language when following up on claims. You will likely not need to know exactly how these are grouped. However, if the clearinghouse or payer

Table 4 *HIPAA Supporting Code Sets*

Adjustment Reason Code	Discipline Type Code	Product/Service Procedure Code
Agency Qualifier Code	Employment Status Code	Prognosis Code
Amount Qualifier Code	Entity Identifier Code	Provider Code
Ambulatory Patient Group Code	Exception Code	Provider Organization Code
Attachment Report Type Code	Facility Type Code	Provider Specialty Certification Code
Attachment Transmission Code	Functional Status Code	Provider Specialty Code
Claim Adjustment Group Code	Hierarchical Child Code	Record Format Code
Claim Filing Indicator Code	Hierarchical Level Code	Reject Reason Code
Claim Frequency Code	Hierarchical Structure Code	Related-Causes Code
Claim Payment Remark Code	Immunization Status Code	Service Type Code
Claim Submission Reason Code	Immunization Type Code	Ship/Delivery or Calendar Pattern Code
Code List Qualifier Code	Individual Relationship Code	Ship/Delivery Pattern Time Code
Condition Codes	Information Release Code	Student Status Code
Contact Function Code	Insurance Type Code	Supporting Document Response Code
Contract Code	Measurement Reference ID Code	Surgical Procedure Code
Contract Type Code	Medicare Assignment Code	Transaction Set Identifier Code
Credit/Debit Flag Code	Nature of Condition Code	Transaction Set Purpose Code
Currency Code	Non-Visit Code	Unit or Basis Measurement Code
Disability Type Code	Note Reference Code	Version Identification Code
	Nutrient Admin Method Code	X-Ray Availability Indicator Code
	Nutrient Admin Technique Code	
	Place of Service Code	
	Policy Compliance Code	

Table 5	Data Grouping in 837P Standard Transaction Format

LEVEL	INFORMATION
High-Level Information: Applies to the entire claim and reflects data pertaining to the billing provider, subscriber, and patient.	Billing/Pay to Provider Information Subscriber/Patient Information Payer Information
Claim-Level Information: Applies to the entire claim and all service lines and is applicable to most claims.	Claim Information Specialty
Specialty Claim–Level Information: Applies to specific claim types.	
Service Line–Level Information: Applies to specific procedure or service that is rendered and is applicable to most claims.	Service Line Information
Specialty Service Line–Level Information: Applies to specific claim types. Required data is only required for the specific claim type.	Specialty Service Line Information
Other Information	Coordination of Benefits (COB) Repriced Claim/Line Credit/Debit Information Clearinghouse/ VAN Tracking

states that you have an invalid item at the "High Level," you will need to understand that it could be incomplete or erroneous information pertaining to the provider, subscriber, or payer (Table 5).

A "friendlier" way to understand this new stream-of-data format is to address a "crosswalk" between the legacy CMS-1500 and the 837P (Table 6; note that dates on HIPAA transactions will be in the format YYYYMMDD [20030806]). Refer to the sample Health Insurance Claim Form.

Standard unique identifiers. The use of standard unique identifiers will improve efficiency in the management of health care by simplifying administration systems. This will enable the efficient electronic transmission of certain health information used across the industry.

- *Standard Unique Employer Identifier* (use EIN to identify employers; compliance by July 30, 2004). The EIN will be used to identify employers rather than inputting the actual name of the company. Employers can use their EINs to identify themselves in transactions involving premium payments to health plans on behalf of their employees or to identify themselves or other employers as the source or receiver of information about eligibility. Employers can also use EINs to identify themselves in transactions when enrolling or disenrolling employees in a health plan.

Text continues on p. 30

PLEASE
DO NOT
STAPLE
IN THIS
AREA

CARRIER

HEALTH INSURANCE CLAIM FORM

PICA | | | | | PICA

1. MEDICARE	MEDICAID	CHAMPUS	CHAMPVA	GROUP HEALTH PLAN	FECA BLK LUNG	OTHER	1a. INSURED'S I.D. NUMBER	(FOR PROGRAM IN ITEM 1)
1 (Medicare #)	(Medicaid #)	(Sponsor's SSN)	(VA File #)	(SSN or ID)	(SSN)	(ID)	**2**	

2. PATIENT'S NAME (Last Name, First Name, Middle Initial)	3. PATIENT'S BIRTH DATE MM DD YY SEX	4. INSURED'S NAME (Last Name, First Name, Middle Initial)
3-4-5-6	**7** M **8** F	**9-10-11-12**

5. PATIENT'S ADDRESS (No., Street)	6. PATIENT RELATIONSHIP TO INSURED	7. INSURED'S ADDRESS (No., Street)
13-14	Self **19-20** Spouse Child Other	**21-22**

CITY	STATE	8. PATIENT STATUS	CITY	STATE
15	**16**	Single Married Other **27-28-29-30-31**	**23**	**24**

ZIP CODE	TELEPHONE (Include Area Code)		ZIP CODE	TELEPHONE (INCLUDE AREA CODE)
17	( ) **18**	Employed Full-Time Student Part-Time Student	**25**	( ) **26**

9. OTHER INSURED'S NAME (Last Name, First Name, Middle Initial)	10. IS PATIENT'S CONDITION RELATED TO:	11. INSURED'S POLICY GROUP OR FECA NUMBER
32-33-34-35	**41**	**46**

a. OTHER INSURED'S POLICY OR GROUP NUMBER	a. EMPLOYMENT? (CURRENT OR PREVIOUS)	a. INSURED'S DATE OF BIRTH MM DD YY SEX
36	**42** YES NO	**47** M **48** F

b. OTHER INSURED'S DATE OF BIRTH MM DD YY SEX	b. AUTO ACCIDENT? PLACE (State)	b. EMPLOYER'S NAME OR SCHOOL NAME
37 M **38** F	**43** YES NO **44**	**49**

c. EMPLOYER'S NAME OR SCHOOL NAME	c. OTHER ACCIDENT?	c. INSURANCE PLAN NAME OR PROGRAM NAME
39	**45** YES NO	**50**

d. INSURANCE PLAN NAME OR PROGRAM NAME	10d. RESERVED FOR LOCAL USE	d. IS THERE ANOTHER HEALTH BENEFIT PLAN?
40		YES **51** NO *If yes, return to and complete item 9 a-d.*

PATIENT AND INSURED INFORMATION

READ BACK OF FORM BEFORE COMPLETING & SIGNING THIS FORM.

12. PATIENT'S OR AUTHORIZED PERSON'S SIGNATURE I authorize the release of any medical or other information necessary to process this claim. I also request payment of government benefits either to myself or to the party who accepts assignment below.

SIGNED **52-53** DATE

13. INSURED'S OR AUTHORIZED PERSON'S SIGNATURE I authorize payment of medical benefits to the undersigned physician or supplier for services described below.

SIGNED **54**

14. DATE OF CURRENT: ILLNESS (First symptom) OR INJURY (Accident) OR PREGNANCY(LMP) MM DD YY	15. IF PATIENT HAS HAD SAME OR SIMILAR ILLNESS. GIVE FIRST DATE MM DD YY	16. DATES PATIENT UNABLE TO WORK IN CURRENT OCCUPATION MM DD YY MM DD YY
55-56-57	**58**	FROM **59** TO **60**

17. NAME OF REFERRING PHYSICIAN OR OTHER SOURCE	17a. I.D. NUMBER OF REFERRING PHYSICIAN	18. HOSPITALIZATION DATES RELATED TO CURRENT SERVICES MM DD YY MM DD YY
61	**62**	FROM **63** TO **64**

19. RESERVED FOR LOCAL USE	20. OUTSIDE LAB? $ CHARGES
65	YES **66** NO **67**

21. DIAGNOSIS OR NATURE OF ILLNESS OR INJURY. (RELATE ITEMS 1,2,3 OR 4 TO ITEM 24E BY LINE)

1. **68**   3. **70**

2. **69**   4. **71**

22. MEDICAID RESUBMISSION CODE	ORIGINAL REF. NO.
72	**73**

23. PRIOR AUTHORIZATION NUMBER

74

24. A DATE(S) OF SERVICE From / To MM DD YY MM DD YY	B Place of Service	C Type of Service	D PROCEDURES, SERVICES, OR SUPPLIES (Explain Unusual Circumstances) CPT/HCPCS	MODIFIER	E DIAGNOSIS CODE	F $ CHARGES	G DAYS OR UNITS	H EPSDT Family Plan	I EMG	J COB	K RESERVED FOR LOCAL USE
75 **76**	**77**	**78**	**79**	**80-81**	**82-83-84-85**	**86**	**87**	**88**	**89**	**90**	**91**

PHYSICIAN OR SUPPLIER INFORMATION

25. FEDERAL TAX I.D. NUMBER SSN EIN	26. PATIENT'S ACCOUNT NO.	27. ACCEPT ASSIGNMENT? (For govt. claims, see back)	28. TOTAL CHARGE	29. AMOUNT PAID	30. BALANCE DUE
92-93	**94**	YES NO **95**	$ **96**	$ **97**	$ **98**

31. SIGNATURE OF PHYSICIAN OR SUPPLIER INCLUDING DEGREES OR CREDENTIALS (I certify that the statements on the reverse apply to this bill and are made a part thereof.)	32. NAME AND ADDRESS OF FACILITY WHERE SERVICES WERE RENDERED (If other than home or office)	33. PHYSICIAN'S, SUPPLIER'S BILLING NAME, ADDRESS, ZIP CODE & PHONE #
SIGNED **99** DATE **100**	**101 thru 106; 108 thru 115**	**116-117-118-119-120-121-122** PIN# **123** GRP# **124**

(APPROVED BY AMA COUNCIL ON MEDICAL SERVICE 8/88)   **PLEASE PRINT OR TYPE**   APPROVED OMB-0938-0008 FORM CMS-1500 (12-90),   FORM RRB-1500,
APPROVED OMB-1215-0055 FORM OWCP-1500,   APPROVED OMB-0720-0001 (CHAMPUS)

Table 6 *Comparison of CMS-1500 and 837P*

Ref. # on CMS	CMS-1500 Box #	CMS-1500 Box Name	837P Data Element #	837P Data Element Name
1	1	Government Program	66	Identification Code Qualifier
2	1a	Insured ID number	67	Subscriber Primary Identifier
3-4-5-6	2	Patients name L, F, MI	1035	Patient Last Name
			1036	Patient First Name
			10.37	Patient Middle Name
			1039	Patient Name Suffix
7	3	Patient Date of Birth	1251	Patient Date of Birth
8	3	Sex	1068	Patient Gender Code
9-10-11-12	4	Insured Name L, F, MI	1035	Patient Last Name
			1036	Patient First Name
			1037	Patient Middle Name
			1039	Patient Name Suffix
13-14	5	Patient Address	166	Patient Address Line
			166	Patient Address Line
15	5	City	19	Patient City Name
16	5	State	156	Patient State Code
17	5	Zip	116	Patient Postal Zone or Zip Code
18	5	Telephone		**NOT USED in 837P**
19-20	6	Patient relationship to Insured, Self, Spouse	1069	Individual Relationship Code
21-22	7	Insured Address	166	Subscriber Address Line
			166	Subscriber Address Line
23	7	City	19	Subscriber City Name
24	7	State	156	State Code
25	7	Zip Code	116	Subscriber Postal Zone or Zip Code

Line	Box	Description	Element	HIPAA 837P Field
26	7	Telephone		NOT USED in 837P
27-28-29-30-31	8	Patient Status Single, Married	1069	Individual Relationship Code
	8	Other	1069	Individual Relationship Code
	8	Employed		NOT USED in 837P
	8	Full-time Student		NOT USED in 837P
	9	Part-time Student		NOT USED in 837P
32-33-34-35	9	Other Insured's Name L, F, MI	1035	Other Insured Last Name
			1036	Other Insured First Name
			1037	Other Insured Middle Name
			1039	Other Insured Name Suffix
36	9a	Other insured Policy or Group Number	93	Other Insured Group Name
37	9b	Other insured date of birth	1251	Other Insured Birth Date
38	9b	Sex	1068	Other Insured Gender Code
39	9c	Employer's name or school name		NOT USED in 837P
40	9d	Insurance plan name or program name	93	Other insured group name
41	10	Is patient's condition related to:		Related causes information:
42	10a	Employment (current or previous)	1362	Related causes code
43	10b	Auto Accident	1362	Related causes code
44	10b	Place (state)	156	Auto accident state or province code
45	10c	Other Accident	1362	Related causes code
46	11	Insured's Policy Group or FECA number		
47	11a	Insured's Date of Birth	1251	Subscriber's birth date
48	11a	Sex	1068	Subscriber gender code
49	11b	Employer's name or school name		NOT USED in 837P
50	11c	Insurance plan name or program name	93	Other insured group name
51	11d	Is there another health benefit plan	98	Entity identifier code

Continued

Data from MEDEXTEND.

Table 6 Comparison of CMS-1500 and 837P—cont'd

Ref. # on CMS	CMS-1500 Box #	CMS-1500 Box Name	837P Data Element #	837P Data Element Name
52-53	12	Patient's or authorized person's signature (and date)	1363	Release of information code
54	13	Insured's or authorized person's signature	1351	Patient Signature source code
			1073	Benefits assignment certification indicator
55-56-57	14	Date of current: Illness, Injury, Pregnancy (LMP)	1251	Initial treatment date
58	15	If patient has had same or similar illness, give first date	1251	Accident date
			1251	LMP
			1251	Similar illness or symptom date
59	16	Dates patient unable to work in current occupation: From	1251	Last worked date
60	16	To	1251	Work return date
61	17	Name of Referring Physician or other source		
62	17a	ID number of referring physician		
63	18	Hospitalization dates related to current services: From	1251	Related hospitalization
64	18	To	1251	Related hospitalization discharge date
65	19	Reserved for local use		
66	20	Outside Lab?		
67	20	$ Charges		
68	21	Diagnosis or nature of illness or injury, 1	1271	Diagnosis code
69	21	2	1271	Diagnosis code
70	21	3	1271	Diagnosis code
71	21	4	1271	Diagnosis code

No.	Box	Field	Ref. No.	837P Field
72	22	Medicaid Resubmission code	127	NOT USED in 837P
73	22	Original ref. No.	127	Claim original reference number
74	23	Prior authorization number	1251	Prior Authorization number
75	24A	Dates of service: From MM DD YY	1251	Order Date
76	24A	To MM DD YY	1331	Order Date
77	24B	Place of Service		Place of Service Code
78	24C	Type of Service		NOT REQUIRED in 837P
79	24D	Procedures, services, or supplies CPT/HCPCS	234	Procedure code
80-81	24D	Modifier	1339	Procedure Modifier
			1339	Procedure Modifier
			1339	Procedure Modifier
82-83-84-85	24E	Diagnosis Code	1328	Diagnosis code pointer
				Diagnosis code pointer
				Diagnosis code pointer
				Diagnosis code pointer
86	24F	$ Charges	782	Line item charge amount
87	24G	Days or units	380	Service unit count
88	24H	EPSDT Family Plan	1366	Special program indicator
89	24I	EMG	1073	Emergency indicator
90	24J	COB		
91	24K	Reserved for local use	127	Rendering provider Secondary Identifier
92	25	Federal Tax ID Number	67	Rendering provider Identifier
93	25	SSN, EIN	66	Identification code qualifier
94	26	Patient's Account No.	1028	Patient account number
95	27	Accept Assignment	1359	Medicare assignment code
96	28	Total charge	782	Total claim charge amount
97	29	Amount Paid	782	Patient amount paid
98	30	Balance Due		

Continued

Data from MEDEXTEND.

Table 6 *Comparison of CMS-1500 and 837P—cont'd*

Ref. # on CMS	CMS-1500 Box #	CMS-1500 Box Name	837P Data Element #	837P Data Element Name
99-100	31	Signature of Physician or supplier (and date)	1073	Provider or supplier signature indicator
101-106; 108-115	32	Name and address of facility where services were rendered	1035	Laboratory or facility name
			166	Laboratory or facility address line
			19	Laboratory or facility city
			156	Laboratory facility state or province code
			116	Laboratory or facility postal zone or zip code
			OR	
			1036	Submitter first name
			1035	Billing provider last or organizational name
			1036	Billing provider first name
			166	Billing provider address line
			166	Billing provider address line
			19	Billing provider city name
			156	Billing provider state or province code

116-122	33	Physicians' suppliers billing name, address, zip code, & phone number	116	Billing provider postal zone or zip code
			1035	Billing provider last or organization name
			1036	Billing provider first name
			166	Billing provider address line
			166	Billing provider address line
			19	Billing provider city name
			156	Billing provider state or province code
			116	Billing provider postal zone or zip code
123	33	Pin #	127	Billing provider additional identifier
124	33	GRP #	67	Billing provider identifier

Data from MEDEXTEND.

- *Standard Unique Health Care Provider Identifier.* Compliance is required by May 23, 2005. This is a 9-position numeric identifier followed by one numeric digit check for the health care provider.

- *Standard Unique Health Plan Identifier.* Proposed Rule estimated to publish November 2004.

- *Standard Unique Patient Identifier.* The intention to create a standard for a uniform patient identifier prompted protest among public interest groups, who saw a universal identifier as a civil liberties threat. Therefore the issue of a universal Patient Identifier is on hold indefinitely.

Corrective Action Plan. CMS has implemented a Corrective Action Plan to address issues of non compliance in regard to TCS. Details at this time are forthcoming and will be available at the CMS website: http://www.cms.gov.

Security Rule: Administrative, Physical, and Technical Safeguards

Security measures encompass all the administrative, physical, and technical safeguards in an information system. The Security Rule addresses only *electronic* protected health information (**ePHI**), but the concept of protecting PHI that will become ePHI makes attention to security for the entire office important. The Security Rule is divided into three main sections: administrative safeguards, technical safeguards and physical safeguards.

Administrative safeguards prevent unauthorized use or disclosure of PHI through administrative actions and P&P to manage the selection, development, implementation, and maintenance of security measures to protect ePHI. These management controls guard data integrity, confidentiality, and availability and include the following:

- Information access controls authorize each employee's physical access to PHI. This is management of password and access for separate employees that restricts their access to records in accordance with their responsibility in the healthcare organization. For example, the medical records clerk who has authorization to retrieve medical records will likely not have access to billing records located on the computer.

- Internal audits allow the ability to review who has had access to PHI to ensure that there is no intentional or accidental inappropriate access, in both the practice management software system and the paper records or charges.

- Risk analysis and management is a process that assesses the privacy and security risks of various safeguards and the cost in losses if those safeguards are not in place. This process is newly introduced into healthcare compliance and each organization must evaluate their vulnerabilities and the associated risks and decide how to mitigate those risks. Reasonable safeguards must be implemented to protect against known risks.

- Termination procedures should be formally documented in the P&P manual and include terminating the employee's access to PHI. Other procedures would likely include changing office security pass codes, deleting user access to computer systems, deleting terminated employee's e-mail account, collecting any access cards or keys.

Technical safeguards are technological controls in place to protect and control access to information on computers in the health care organization and include the following:

- Access controls consist of user-based access (system set up to place limitations on access to data tailored to each staff member) and role-based access (limitations created for each job category, e.g. scheduling, billing, clinical).

- Audit controls keep track of log-ins to the computer system, administrative activity, and changes to data. This includes changing passwords, deleting user accounts, or creating a new user.

- Automatic log-offs prevent unauthorized users from accessing a computer when it is left unattended. The computer system or software program should automatically log-off after a predetermined period of inactivity. Your office's practice management software may have this useful feature; if not, the feature may be temporarily mimicked using a screen-saver and password.

- Each user should have a unique identifier or "username" and an unshared, undisclosed password to log into any computer with access to PHI. Identifying each unique user allows the functions of auditing and access controls to be implemented. Other authentication techniques involve more sophisticated devices, such as a magnetic card or fingerprints. You likely will be dealing only with a password in your organization. Passwords for all users should be changed on a regular basis and should never be common names or words.

- *Physical safeguards* also prevent unauthorized access to PHI. These physical measures and P&P protect a covered entity's electronic information systems and related buildings and equipment from natural and environmental hazards and unauthorized intrusion. Appropriate and reasonable physical safeguards should include the following:

- Media and equipment controls are documented P&P regarding the management of media and equipment containing the PHI. Typical safeguard policies include how the organization handles the retention, removal, and disposal of paper records, as well as the recycling of computers and destruction of obsolete data disks or software programs containing PHI.

- Physical access controls limit unauthorized access to areas where equipment is stored as well as medical charts. Locks on doors are the most common type of control.

- Secure workstation locations minimize the possibility of unauthorized viewing of PHI. This includes making sure that password-protected screensavers are in use on computers when unattended and that desk drawers are locked.

Application to Practice Setting

HIPAA affects all areas of the health care office, from the reception area to the provider. In conjunction with being educated and trained in job responsibilities, every staff member must be educated about HIPAA and trained in the P&P pertinent to the organization.

Best practices are strategies for constantly improving productivity and service. Best practices are deployed and produce demonstrable results that meet federal and state mandates and the practice's objectives. Results and benefits are documented and measured periodically to assess for efficiency in terms of dollars, time, and other resource costs. "Best" does not mean 'most,' as in "most organizations do things this way" or "the most expensive solution."

Best practice is a way to perform in the most efficient and effective manner for your particular organizational environment. In the revenue or claims cycle, for example, your office may have all charges for services posted by Thursday afternoon and may not see patients on Fridays. Your organization may employ a "best practice" of generating and transmitting claims every Friday afternoon. This is efficient because there are no distractions with patient appointments, and the routine of every Friday keeps claims filed in a timely manner. This leads to a positive cash flow.

Reasonable safeguards are measurable solutions based on accepted standards that are implemented and periodically monitored to demonstrate that the office is in compliance. Reasonable efforts must be made to limit the use or disclosure of PHI. If you are the front desk receptionist and you close the privacy glass between your desk and the waiting area when you are making a call to a patient, this is a reasonable safeguard to prevent others in the waiting room from overhearing.

Incidental uses and disclosures are permissible under HIPAA only when reasonable safeguards or precautions have been implemented to prevent misuse or inappropriate disclosure of PHI. When incidental uses and disclosures result from failure to apply reasonable safeguards or adhere to the minimum necessary standard, the Privacy Rule has been violated. If you are in the reception area and you close the privacy glass when having a confidential conversation, and you are still overheard by an individual in the waiting room, this would be "incidental." You have applied a reasonable safeguard to prevent this from happening.

Guidelines for HIPAA privacy compliance. As a health care provider, you will likely answer the telephone and speak during the course of your business, and there will be questions about what you can and cannot say. Reasonable and appropriate safeguards must be taken to ensure that all confidential health information in your office is protected from unauthorized and inappropriate access, including both verbal and written forms.

1. Consider that conversations occurring throughout the office could be overheard. The reception area and waiting room are often linked, and it is easy to hear the scheduling of appointments and exchange of confidential information. It is necessary to observe areas and maximize efforts to avoid unauthorized disclosures. Simple and affordable

precautions include using privacy glass at the front desk and having conversations away from settings where other patients or visitors are present. Health care providers can move their dictation stations away from patient areas or wait until no patients are present before dictating. Phone conversations by providers in front of patients, even in emergency situations, should be avoided. Providers and staff must use their best professional judgment.

2. Be sure to check in the patient medical record and in your computer system to see if there are any special instructions for contacting the patient regarding scheduling or reporting test results. Follow these requests as agreed by the office.

3. Patient sign-in sheets *are* permissible, but limit the information you request when a patient signs in, and change it periodically during the day. A sign-in sheet must not contain information such as reason for visit because some providers specialize in treating patients with sensitive issues. Showing that a particular individual has an appointment with your practice may pose a breach of patient confidentiality.

4. Make sure you have patients sign a form acknowledging receipt of the NPP. The NPP allows you to release the patient's confidential information for billing and other purposes. If your practice has other confidentiality statements and policies besides HIPAA mandates, these must be reviewed to ensure they meet HIPAA requirements.

5. Formal policies for transferring and accepting outside PHI must address how your office keeps this information confidential. When using courier services, billing services, transcription services, or e-mail, you must ensure that transferring PHI is done in a secure and compliant manner.

6. Computers are used for a variety of administrative functions, including scheduling, billing, and managing medical records. Computers typically are present at the reception area. Keep the computer screen turned so that viewing is restricted to authorized staff. Screensavers should be used to prevent unauthorized viewing or access. The computer should automatically log off the user after a period of being idle, requiring the staff member to reenter their password.

7. Keep your username and password confidential, and change it often. Do not share this information. An authorized staff member such as the PO will have administrative access to reset your password if you lose it or if someone discovers it. Also, practice management software can track users and follow their activity. Do not set yourself up by giving out your password. Safeguards include password protection for electronic data and storing paper records securely.

8. Safeguard your work area; do not place notes with confidential information in areas that are easy to view by nonstaff. Cleaning services will access your building, usually after business hours; ensure that you safeguard PHI.

9. Place medical record charts face down at reception areas so the patient's name is not exposed to other patients or visitors to your office. Also, when placing medical records on the door of an examination room, turn the chart so that identifying information faces the door. If you keep medical charts in the office on countertops or in receptacles, it is your duty to ensure that nonstaff persons will not access the records. Handling and storing medical records will certainly change because of HIPAA guidelines.

10. Do not post the health care provider's schedule in areas viewable by nonstaff individuals. The schedules are often posted for professional staff convenience, but this may be a breach in patient confidentiality.

11. Fax machines should not be placed in patient examination rooms or in any reception area where nonstaff persons may view incoming or sent documents. Only staff members should have access to the faxes.

12. If you open your office mail or take phone calls pertaining to medical record requests, direct these issues to the appropriate staff member.

13. If you are involved in coding and billing, be sure to recognize, learn, and use HIPAA TCS.

14. Send all privacy-related questions or concerns to the appropriate staff member.

15. Immediately report any suspected or known improper behavior to your supervisor or the PO so that the issue may be documented and investigated.

16. If you have questions, contact your supervisor or the PO.

Health care organizations face challenges in implementing the HIPAA requirements; do not let these overwhelm you. Your office is required to take reasonable steps to build protections specific to your health care organization. Compliance is an ongoing endeavor involving teamwork. Understand your office's established P&P. Monitor your own activities to ensure you are following the required procedures. Do not take shortcuts when your actions involve patient privacy and security.

Be alert to other activities in your office. Help your co-workers change work habits that do not comply with HIPAA. Do not ignore unauthorized uses and disclosures of PHI, and do not allow unauthorized persons to access data. You have an obligation to your employer and the patients you serve.

Consequences of Noncompliance with HIPAA

The prosecution of HIPAA crimes is handled by different governing bodies. HHS handles issues regarding TCS and security. Complaints can be filed against a covered entity for not complying with these rules. The OCR oversees privacy issues and complaints, referring criminal issues to the Office of Inspector General (OIG). The OIG provides the workup for referral cases, which may involve the FBI and other agencies.

Serious civil and criminal penalties apply for HIPAA noncompliance. General noncompliance with the privacy, security and transaction regulations result in a $100 fine per violation and up to $25,000 per person for identical violations in a given calendar year. Specific to the Privacy Rule is a $50,000 fine and imprisonment for 1 year if one knowingly obtains or discloses IIHI. The person who obtains or discloses such health information under false pretenses is subject to a $100,000 fine. If one obtains or discloses PHI with the intent to sell, transfer, or use it for commercial advantage, personal gain, or malicious harm, a maximum fine of $250,000 and up to 10 years' imprisonment may be applied.

OFFICE OF INSPECTOR GENERAL

The mission of the OIG is to safeguard the health and welfare of the beneficiaries of HHS programs and to protect the integrity of HHS programs (Medicare and Medicaid). The OIG was established to identify and eliminate fraud, abuse, and waste and "to promote efficiency and economy in departmental operations." HIPAA legislation has radically changed the focus and mission within OIG. HIPAA pushed OIG into a new era, guaranteeing funding for the OIG programs and mandating initiatives to protect the integrity of all health care programs. The OIG undertakes nationwide audits, as well as investigations and inspections to review the claim submission processes of providers and reimbursement patterns of the programs. Recommendations are made to the HHS Secretary and the U.S. Congress on correcting problematic areas addressed in the federal programs. According to the OIG:

> Efforts to combat fraud were consolidated and strengthened under Public Law 104-191, the Health Insurance Portability and Accountability Act of 1996 (HIPAA). The Act established a comprehensive program to combat fraud committed against all health plans, both public and private. The legislation required the establishment of a national Health Care Fraud and Abuse Control Program (HCFAC), under the joint direction of the Attorney General and the Secretary of the Department of Health and Human Services (HHS) acting through the Department's Inspector General (HHS/OIG). The HCFAC program is designed to coordinate Federal, State, and local law enforcement activities with respect to health care fraud and abuse. The Act requires HHS and DOJ [Department of Justice] to detail in an Annual Report the amounts deposited and appropriated to the Medicare Trust Fund, and the source of such deposits.

Health care providers must be aware of the potential liabilities when submitting claims for payment that are deemed to be "fraudulent" or inappropriate by the government. The government may impose significant financial and administrative penalties when health care claims are not appropriately submitted, including criminal prosecution against the offending party. Fraud, according to the OIG, can result from deliberate unethical behavior or simply from mistakes and miscues that cause excessive reimbursement. The OIG is the professional health care provider's (and their agents') "partner" in fighting fraud and abuse.

Compliance Program Guidance recommendations from the OIG must be the guiding principle of a health care practice in regard to the potential for unethical behavior or the mistakes that may occur within the organization. The *Individual and Small Group Physician Practices* and *Compliance Program Guidance for Third-Party Medical Billing Companies* are two publications in a series for the health care industry that provides guidance and acceptable principles for business operations.

If you are involved in the claims-processing procedures in your organization, note the importance and urgency in following the legal and ethical path when performing your duties. Your "honest mistake" could lead to a situation that puts the health care provider at risk for investigation of fraud, waste, or abuse.

Fraud and Abuse Laws

Fraud can occur when deception is used in a claim submission to obtain payment from the payer. Individuals who knowingly, willfully, and intentionally submit false information to benefit themselves or others commit fraud. Fraud can also be interpreted from mistakes that result in excessive reimbursement. No proof of "specific intent to defraud" is required for fraud to be considered.

Abuse occurs when a health care organization practices behavior that is not indicative of sound medical or fiscal activity.

Federal False Claims Act (31 US Code §3729-33). "A false claim is a claim for payment for services or supplies that were not provided specifically as presented or for which the provider is otherwise not entitled to payment.". Presenting a claim for an item or service based on a code known to result in greater payment or submitting a claim for services not medically necessary is also a violation of the False Claims Act (FCA). The government uses the FCA as a primary enforcement tool.

Although no proof of specific intent to defraud is required, liability can occur when a person knowingly presents or causes to present such a claim or makes, uses, or causes a false record or statement to have a false or fraudulent claim paid or approved by the federal government.

Qui Tam "Whistleblower." Qui Tam in the FCA provisions allows a private citizen to bring a civil action suit for a violation on behalf of the federal government. This involves fraud by government contractors and other entities who receive or use government funds. The Qui Tam "whistleblower" shares in any money recovered.

Civil Monetary Penalties Law (42 US Code §320a-27a). The U.S. Congress enacted the Civil Monetary Penalty (CMP) statute to provide administrative remediation to combat health care fraud and abuse. The HIPAA's Final Rule includes civil monetary penalties when there is a pattern of upcoded claims or billing for medically unnecessary services. CMP imposes civil money penalties and assessments against a person or organization for making false or improper claims against any federal health care program.

Criminal False Claims Act (18 US Code). The Criminal False Claims Act did not apply specifically to the health care industry before HIPAA. HIPAA amendments to the criminal code include the following:

- **Theft or Embezzlement (18 US Code §669).** This law brings fines and imprisonment against any individual who "knowingly and willfully embezzles, steals, or otherwise without authority converts to the use of any person other than the rightful owner, or intentionally misapplies any of the moneys, funds, securities, premiums, credits, property, or other assets of a health care benefit program." This law does not just affect Medicare and Medicaid programs.

- **False Statement Relating to Health Care Matters (18 US Code §1035).** Any individual who knowingly and willfully "falsifies, conceals, or covers up by any trick, scheme, or device a material fact; or makes any materially false, fictitious, or fraudulent statements or representations, or makes or uses any materially false writing or document knowing the same to contain any materially false, fictitious, or fraudulent statement or entry, in connection with the delivery of or payment for health care benefits, items, or services" is subject to fines and imprisonment.

- **Health Care Fraud (18 US Code §1347).** Any individual who knowingly and willfully "executes, or attempts to execute, a scheme or artifice to defraud any health care benefit program; or to obtain, by means of false or fraudulent pretenses, representations, or promises, any of the money or property owned by, or under the custody or control of, any health care benefit program, in connection with the delivery of or payment for health care benefits, items, or services" is subject to fines and imprisonment. If seriously bodily injury or even death occurs, the person may face life imprisonment.

- **Obstruction of Criminal Investigations of Health Care Offenses (18 US Code §1518).** An individual is subject to fines and imprisonment when the person "willfully prevents, obstructs, misleads, delays or attempts to prevent, obstruct, mislead, or delay the communication of information or records relating to a violation of a Federal health care offense to a criminal investigator."

Stark Laws (42 US Code §1395). Stark Laws prohibit the submission of claims for "designated services" or referral of patients if the referring physician has a "financial relationship" with the entity that provides the services. Originally named "Stark I," this law pertained only to clinical laboratories. Stark Laws carry exceptions, so it is important to understand the referral processes and in-office ancillary services used by your health care organization.

Anti-Kickback Statute. According to CMS, discounts, rebates, or other reductions in price may violate the Anti-Kickback Statute because such arrangements induce the purchase of items or services payable by Medicare or Medicaid. However, some arrangements are clearly permissible if they fall within a "safe harbor." One safe harbor protects certain discounting practices. For purposes of this safe harbor, a "discount" is the reduction in the amount a seller charges a buyer for a good or service based on an "arms-length" transaction. In addition, to be protected under the discount safe harbor, the discount must apply to the original item or service purchased or furnished; that is, a discount cannot be applied to the purchase of a different good or service than the one on which the discount was earned. A "rebate" is defined as a discount that is not given at the time of sale. A "buyer" is the individual or entity responsible for submitting a claim for the item or service that is payable by the Medicare or Medicaid programs. A "seller" is the individual or entity who offers the discount.

Safe Harbors. Safe harbors specify various business and service arrangements that are protected from prosecution under the Anti-Kickback Statute. These include certain investments, care in underserved areas, and other arrangements.

Additional laws and compliance. Other laws pertaining to fraud and abuse include the Federal Deposit Insurance Corporation (FDIC) Mail and Wire Fraud provisions, as follows:

- **§1341. Frauds and swindles.** An individual is subject to both fines and imprisonment when having "devised or intending to devise any scheme or artifice to defraud, or for obtaining money or property by means of false or fraudulent pretenses" by use of the U.S. Postal Service, whether sent by or delivered to the Postal Service.

- **§1343. Fraud by wire, radio, or television.** An individual will be fined and/or imprisoned "for obtaining money or property by means of false or fraudulent pretenses, representations, or promises, transmits or causes to be transmitted by means of wire, radio, or television communication."

The U.S. government is clearly committed to the investigation and prosecution of health care fraud. As with HIPAA policies and procedures, it is imperative that health care entities develop their own compliance program to identify and prevent fraud.

Government Strategies to Reduce Health Care Fraud

Health Care Fraud and Abuse Program. HCFAP has created a national fraud and abuse program by coordinating efforts of enforcement agencies at local, state, and federal levels.

Operation Restore Trust. Launched in 1995, Operation Restored Trust (ORT) was designed to coordinate the activities of the OIG along with CMS and other HHS entities in identifying and preventing fraud. An established hotline (1-800-HHS-TIPS) for the public allows reporting issues that might indicate fraud, abuse, or waste. ORT has been successful due to planning with the Department of Justice (DOJ) and other law enforcement agencies, training state and local organizations to detect fraud and abuse, and implementing statistical methods to identify providers for audits and investigations.

Medicare Integrity Program. The goal of the Medicare Integrity Program (MIP) is to identify and reduce Medicare overpayments through a series of audits and reviews of provider claims and cost report data. Initiatives of MIP include identifying plan beneficiaries with additional insurance and educating health care providers. Program integrity contractors help expand the scope of the MIP. This endeavor has recovered several billions of dollars in the fight against fraud waste and abuse in the Medicare program.

Correct Coding Initiative. The Correct Coding Initiative (CCI) was developed to detect improperly coded claims through the use of computer edits. Services that should be grouped together and paid as one item rather than billed separately to obtain higher reimbursement are identified with the computer system.

Increased staffing and expanded penalties for violations. A significant increase in staffing among the OIG, DOJ, and FBI over the past decade has included prosecutors (over 400% increase since 1993) and FBI agents (over 300% since 1993). With additional employees, the industry has seen the promotion of compliance endeavors across the health care sector. Penalties for violations have increased.

Special alerts, bulletins, and guidance documents. Special Fraud Alerts are published by the OIG to alert the industry concerning specific patterns or trends related to fraudulent or abusive activities regarding the Medicare and Medicaid programs. Special Advisory Bulletins report industry practices and arrangements that may implicate fraud and abuse. Other guidance documents include updates, response letters and alerts important to more specifically targeted matters. All notices are available at the OIG website, and you can sign up for their mailing list.

Exclusion Program. According to OIG:

> No program payment will be made for anything that an excluded person furnishes, orders, or prescribes. This payment prohibition applies to the excluded person, anyone who employs or contracts with the excluded person, any hospital or other provider where the excluded person provides services, and anyone else. The exclusion applies regardless of who submits the claims and applies to all administrative and management services furnished by the excluded person.

Excluded persons/facilities are convicted for program-related fraud and patient abuse, actions from licensing boards, and defaulting on Health Education Assistance Loans.

Your health care organization must not conduct business with any health care provider or subcontract with any agent who has been listed as an Excluded Individual. Be sure to check the updated listings at the OIG website.

Compliance Program Guidance for Individual and Small Group Physician Practices

The OIG published the *Individual and Small Group Physician Practices* in September 2000. This guidance recommended by the OIG is voluntary; however, an effective plan reduces the risk of legal action and creates a "good faith" effort in combating fraud, waste, and abuse. A compliance plan requires that a health care practice review all billing processes through audits and establish controls that will correct weaknesses and prevent errors.

A well-designed compliance program can speed the claims-processing cycle; optimize proper payment or claims; minimize billing mistakes; reduce the likelihood of a government audit; avoid conflict with Stark Laws and the Anti-Kickback Statute; show a "good faith" effort that claims will be submitted appropriately; and relay to staff that there is a duty to report mistakes and suspected or known misconduct.

If you are a claims-processing staff member, your organization's claims-processing supervisor should research industry sector program guidance to help with specific concerns regarding the specialty/facility setting. Check the OIG website to view addendums, comments, and drafts of additional compliance guidance subjects. Other program guidance includes the following:

- June 2004: Draft Supplemental Compliance Program Guidance for Hospitals

- April 2003: Guidance for Pharmaceutical Industry

- March 2003: Ambulance Suppliers

- September 2000: Individual and Small Group Physician Practices

- February 2000: Nursing Facilities

- November 1999: Medicare + Choice Organizations

- September 1999: Hospices

- June 1999: Durable Medical Equipment Prosthetics, Orthotics, and Supply Industry

- November 1998: Third-Party Medical Billing Companies

- August 1998: Home Health Agencies

- August 1998: Clinical Laboratories

- February 1998: Hospitals

Increased productivity and decreased penalties with compliance plan. The presence of an OIG compliance program can significantly mitigate imposed penalties in the event of an OIG audit or other discovery of fraudulent billing activities. These P&P can be found in the provider's P&P manual. For those not currently in the role of a Privacy/Security/Compliance Officer, knowledge about P&P as they pertain to both HIPAA and OIG will be invaluable throughout their career.

Because health care providers rely on the expertise of their billing and coding staff to process claims accurately and promptly, they also look to these staff members for advice and guidance. If you are directly involved in this area of your organization, you will likely be expected to understand the complexities of the various laws and regulations governing the medical claims process.

Compliance plans effectively become a "meeting of the minds" among the players; providers, claims-processing staff, and payers all are agreeing to process claims in accordance with shared values. Consider your organization's OIG compliance program as a way to integrate regulatory requirements directly into your claims-processing procedures. OIG views the experienced claims-processing staff as the critical screen for the health care provider's claims. The common denominators in the key benefits identified by OIG are efficiency, consistency, and integrity.

Seven Basic Components of a Compliance Plan

OIG outlines the following seven components of an effective program guidance plan specifically for the individual and small group physician practices:

1. Conducting internal monitoring and auditing.

2. Implementing compliance and practice standards.

3. Designating a compliance officer or contact.

4. Conducting appropriate training and education.

5. Responding appropriately to detected offenses and developing corrective action.

6. Developing open lines of communication.

7. Enforcing disciplinary standards through well-publicized guidelines.

Conducting internal monitoring and auditing. A comprehensive auditing and monitoring program will not eliminate misconduct within an organization but will minimize the risk of fraud and abuse by identifying the risk areas. OIG does not provide a specific set of guidelines on conducting audits or ongoing monitoring. The compliance officer, with the committee's assistance, should identify problem areas and should have established auditing priorities and procedures as part of the organization's compliance program.

Special attention should be made to the risk areas associated with Claims Submission and Processing. Also, a thorough review of the organization's standards and written P&P should be conducted to ensure proper guidelines for complying with state and federal laws and insurance payer requirements.

Implementing compliance and practice standards. Written standards and procedures will address risk areas that an office needs to monitor and follow. Specific risk areas identified by OIG include the following:

- Billing for items or services not rendered or not provided as claimed.

- Submitting claims for equipment, medical supplies, and services that are not reasonable and necessary.

- Double billing resulting in duplicate payment.

- Billing for noncovered services as if covered.

- Knowing misuse of provider identification numbers, which results in improper billing.

- Unbundling, or billing for each component of the service instead of billing or using an all-inclusive code.

- Failure to use coding modifiers properly.

- Clustering.

- Upcoding the level of service provided.

Data from *Federal Register* 65(194):59439, 2000.

In addition to these risk areas, policies should be developed that address the following:

- Reasonable and necessary
- Proper medical documentation
- Federal sentencing guidelines
- Record retention

You should be able to access your organization's P&P manual to review the standards and protocol for these issues involving your practice.

Designating a compliance officer or contact. As with the HIPAA Privacy Officer (PO), the Compliance Officer is the key individual overseeing your organization's compliance program monitoring with the support of the Compliance Committee. Again, as with HIPAA, policies and procedures (P&P) need to be drafted. These established guidelines identify and prevent fraud and abuse activities as described by OIG.

The number of members on your Compliance Committee is not important, and prospective staff members from human resources, claims auditing, billing, legal, and medicine can ensure a comprehensive mix. You may currently participate on your office's Compliance Committee or may be asked to do so in the future. The Compliance Committee acts as a review board. Some committees consist of provider-client office staff and billing company staff. Some committees are simply the provider-client and the billing company staff, or a combination of the provider-client, their practice manager, and the billing company staff. The Committee, empowered by management, legitimizes the compliance strategy within your organization. In addition to possessing professional experience in claims processing and auditing, Committee members will be expected to use good judgment and high integrity to fulfill committee obligations.

Conducting appropriate training and education. Because OIG compliance program guidelines are based on Federal Sentencing Guidelines, significant elements of an effective compliance program involve proper education and training of staff. Every employee and individual who interacts with your health care organization and may be accountable for potential misconduct should be considered in the organization's training sessions.

You should be required to attend training in a "general" compliance training session at least annually. For staff members involved in claims processing (coding and billing), a separate training session should be held to cover internal procedures, federal and state laws regarding fraud and abuse, and specific government and other payer reimbursement policies. Periodic professional courses in continuing education should be available. Coding and billing personnel should receive training at least annually to remain updated on CPT/HCPCS and ICD-9-CM codes for each year. You will attend training either on site, at a remote location, or both.

Effective training can reduce potential errors, penalties, and fines. An educated staff makes fewer errors, reduces your organization's risks, and requires less micromanagement.

Responding appropriately to detected offenses and developing corrective action. When faced with the discovery of an offense or an error, inaction may be interpreted as indifference. This could impose a potential jeopardy to the reputation of the health care provider's practice. Your office should have a process for investigating problems and taking necessary corrective action. Issues that would raise concern include significant change in claims that are rejected; software edits that show pattern of misuse of codes or fees; unusually high volume of charges, payments, or rejections; and notices from insurance payers regarding claims submitted by your office.

You and your fellow staff members should be encouraged to report concerns for any suspected or known misconduct, with an established chain of command in the reporting path. Some incidences of misconduct may violate criminal, civil, or administrative law. Should the situation warrant, the Compliance Officer should report the misconduct promptly to the appropriate government authority.

Report fraud and abuse. Contact the HHS OIG as follows:

- PHONE HOTLINE 800-HHS-TIPS (1-800-447-8477)
- TTY 800-377-4950
- FAX 800-223-8164
- http://oig.hhs.gov/hotline.html

Developing open lines of communication. Effective lines of communication provide a channel for employees to report suspected or known misconduct without immediately resorting to an external agency. In this way your health care organization can resolve issues internally. "Open door" policies ensure an environment where staff members feel secure to ask about the organization's existing P&P and to report questionable activities. Your role as a conscientious employee will allow you to know the steps to take in reporting any suspicious business activity.

You will learn your office's procedure for reporting misconduct. It is important to follow these guidelines to protect your reputation and credibility within the workplace. Depending on the size of the practice, the methods for contacting managerial staff may include anonymous telephone calls through a "hotline" or written report forms.

Enforcing disciplinary standards through well-publicized guidelines. The unfortunate downside to compliance is that misconduct does occur. For this reason, health care organizations must have established disciplinary guidelines and must make these well known to employees and other agents who contract with the organization. We all want to know what will happen if we "make a mistake" and what progressive forms of discipline await situations involving misconduct. Disciplinary standards include the following:

- Verbal warning

- Written warning

- Written reprimand

- Suspension or probation

- Demotion

- Termination of employment

- Restitution of any damages

- Referral to federal agencies for criminal prosecution

Whether the misconduct was intentional or negligent, all levels of employees need to know what is expected of them. Your office must publish this information and disseminate it to all employees.

What to Expect from Your Health Care Practice

Although every health care organization or practice is different in regard to policies and procedures, you now know what to expect in the workplace, as follows:

- Practice Adherence to HIPAA and OIG Mandates and Recommendations

- Privacy/Security/Compliance Officer (even if one person)

- Policy and Procedure Manual

- Employee Training and Education (at least annually and whenever there are changes in business operations that affect staff members directly)

- Complaint and Sanctions Process

Compliance Lessons Learned

You must strongly consider the lessons learned from the privacy, transaction, and security rules in conjunction with OIG compliance recommendations. The most important points are to read your organization's P&P manual and to ask questions about the many aspects of HIPAA or the general operations of your organization. Always use your ethical and "best practice" approach to be an informed and effective employee.

DATA SOURCES AND REFERENCES

American Health Information Management Association
http://www.ahima.org

Centers for Medicare and Medicaid
http://www.cms.gov

HIPAAdocs Corporation
http://www.hipaadocs.com

MEDEXTEND
http://www.medextend.com

Office of Civil Rights
http://www.hhs.gov/ocr/hipaa

Office of Inspector General
http://www.oig.hhs.gov

OIG Compliance Program Guidance for Third-Party Medical Billing Companies, *Federal Register* 63(243):70141, 1998.

OIG Compliance Program for Individual and Small Group Physician Practices, *Federal Register* 65(194):59439, 2000.

Phoenix Health Systems: HIPAA Advisory
http://www.hipaadvisory.com

Workgroup for Electronic Data Interchange
http://www.wedi.org